A Beginner's Guide to ME/CFS

Myalgic Encephalomyelitis (aka CFS, CFS/ME, ME/CFS etc)

Nancy Blake, BA, CQSW
Including recommendations by
Leslie O Simpson, PhD

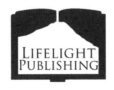
LIFELIGHT
PUBLISHING

Published by Lifelight Publishing 2013
www.lifelightpublishing.com

Cover photo and design by Grainger Graphics

Copyright © Nancy Blake 2013
www.nancyblakealternatives.com

British Library Cataloguing in Publication Data. A catalogue record for this book is available from the British Library.

ISBN: 0-9571817-4-4
ISBN-13: 978-0-9571817-4-8

10 9 8 7 6 5 4 3 2 1

A Beginner's Guide to

Guide to

ME/CFS

TABLE OF CONTENTS

PREAMBLE

I need to thank a reader (who has had ME for several years) and her mother, who looked at this book before publication, and were kind enough to make the effort to read through it all and send me their reactions. In light of their comments I have taken into account the following issues:

For the patient, information needs to be simple and straightforward otherwise the effort to read it is just too much. This point has been made by others.

I hadn't said enough about the symptoms – the suffering – involved in having this illness. Our state has been likened to that of a person in the advanced stages of multiple sclerosis, chronic obstructive pulmonary disorder, or of a person with AIDS three weeks before death. These analogies might give you some idea of what it is like to have ME.

And I had not offered any direct advice for the dedicated (and exhausted!) carers who are keeping us going – even keeping us alive.

I have pointed out the sections that can be skipped, added a brief summary at the end, and included a section in praise of carers: ***You need to know that every single task you do for us can take us closer to the possibility of getting better.***

Finally, we are in a double bind: the more we say about the symptoms, the more we sound like hypochondriacs. It is hard to believe (even for people who have ME!) how long it goes on for, how many different symptoms we get, how much worse we get when we try to overcome it, and how the illness varies, even from hour to hour. (1) You couldn't make it up – and we haven't!

THIS BOOK IS DEDICATED TO YOU, THE READER

Maybe you just got sick. Maybe you've been sick a few times, it lasted a few weeks and you got better, but now it isn't getting better.

You feel like your muscles are just not working properly – you try to walk across the room and you have to lie down to recover. The more you try to do things, the worse it gets. More effort leads to headaches, muscle pains, dizziness, feeling sick. And it isn't just your muscles that aren't working. You can't remember anything for more than three seconds, and the minute anyone starts explaining something to you, your brain just checks out. Not going to do it. Your sleeping pattern has gone to pot, sometimes you have a fever and sometimes you are freezing cold, it's like your body has forgotten how to regulate anything. And just to add to the complications of life with ME, you may have problems with peeing – either you can't, or you have to, all the time. Oh, and you get emotional, quite quickly – but don't let anyone call it hysterical! Anyone who is at the very limit of physical exhaustion, and beyond it, is going to be easily upset – weepy or cross. It's called 'the last straw'! Having ME is *being* at that limit of exhaustion and beyond it – twenty four hours a day, for no apparent reason.

And by the way, you are the farthest thing from a hypochondriac. You've always thrown yourself into things, worked hard, ignored minor injuries and illnesses – you feel pretty contemptuous of people who just give up and don't try to rise above things. You've always ploughed on, no matter what.

So this is pretty frightening. You've never suffered from anxiety or depression, but after a few weeks of this, you are both anxious and depressed, for very good reason. And you are feeling angry at yourself for not being able, this time, to ignore it until it goes away. You expect to get over things, whatever they are, and this is just going on and on and on and on…

You call your doctor, or you get to your doctor somehow. You want a diagnosis, and you want treatment. If this scenario hasn't already happened, let me warn you: your doctor is probably not going to be very happy with you. She or he may just 'not believe in ME', in which case you are likely to get something of a talking to, of the kind that you've already given to yourself on numerous occasions. It goes along the lines of 'There's nothing wrong with you, get over it, stop being silly and stop wasting the doctor's time.' You would like nothing better than for this approach to work, after all, it's what you've always done before. However, when it doesn't, both you and the doctor are likely to get very frustrated.

You may find that your doctor is sympathetic but baffled. However, if he or she follows the NICE Guidelines (2), you will be given a series of routine tests to eliminate other possibilities. If you are given a diagnosis of ME (myalgic encephalomyelitis) or CFS (chronic fatigue syndrome), (or CFS/ME, or ME/CFS) you will learn two things:

1)   Exertion, physical or mental (or emotional stress) but especially just physical exertion will 'exacerbate symptoms' e.g. make you get worse. (You already know this only too well)

2)   The treatments recommended as 'evidence-based' are Cognitive Behaviour Therapy (changing your belief that you have an organic illness) and Graded Exercise Therapy (to get you used to exercising, and get rid of the 'false illness belief' that exercise will make you worse).

Prescribing something which is known to make an illness worse as a treatment for it doesn't make a lot of sense, and patient groups are virtually united in protesting against this. It is the psychiatrists who label ME/CFS as a 'functional somatoform disorder' (3) who are operating from 'false beliefs': there are many 'biomarkers' proving that ME/CFS has a range of physiological effects (4), but, because of the influence of the psychiatric lobby, the NICE Guidelines instruct your doctor not to test for these.

I got sick in the spring of 1986, and I remained very frightened and confused until a friend brought me the article about ME which was published in The Observer, the following June. (5) This article contained an exact description of my illness, including the information that, at that time, there were no clear-cut diagnostic tests, and there was no known cure, except rest. I was terribly relieved. It wasn't going to get worse until I died (as long as I rested), and it wasn't going to kill me. I showed the article to my doctor, who had a hissy-fit because he was 'sure' it was psychological. He referred me to another doctor in the practice (a very sensible woman), who did the routine tests to eliminate anything else and just told me to ask for a sick note when I needed one.

I think your doctor is likely to appreciate your wanting to be as little trouble as possible, and that might improve your chances of getting help at a time when you absolutely need it. For example, help with a sick note, or an application for assistance on the basis of disability, or support when explaining to your employer or your school that you will need special consideration and perhaps modifications to your environment in order to continue despite your illness.

When I first became ill, there were no specialist treatment centres, and almost no one in the medical profession dealing with ME. In recent years, the psychiatric lobby has got funding for specialist centres, the majority of which will practice along the lines recommended by those who adhere to the psychosocial view of ME, offering CBT and GET. (6) If your doctor offers you a referral, it might be wise to do a little research into what kind of treatment they are likely to offer, and proceed with a degree of caution. CBT can be offered in the spirit of helping you to adapt to having a serious physical illness, in which case it could be supportive. GET may encourage very minimal exertion, with sensitive concern not to make you worse. Individual practitioners may be genuinely supportive. If, on the other hand, CBT is intended to persuade you that you don't have a physical illness, and GET is based on the idea that you only imagine exercise will harm you, *these treatments will make you worse*. (7) Try to find out which is on offer, before engaging with a referral to a specialist unit. Members of a local support group might be a useful source of information.

SO WHAT *CAN* YOU DO?

You are not on your own. There are many very well-informed support groups, and groups that are conducting or supporting medical research. It is through these websites that you are likely to get the most helpful information and advice. (At the end of the book you'll find a list, with comments about what they each do best.)

In the meantime: **REST. AND REST. AND REST.**

Master the paradox of ME: The only way to fight ME is to stop fighting.

ME is an upside-down illness. It is an illness that runs against powerful currents of opinion. The widely held view is that taking the paracetamol and carrying on is the right thing to do; mind power can conquer all; and exercise is good for absolutely everything from warts to cancer.

- *Do not take the paracetamol and carry on: Stop!*

- *Mind power cannot conquer all, so use your mind power to learn that the key to recovery is inactivity.*

- *Exercise will make you worse.*

- *More exercise will make you very much worse for very much longer.*

- *Even more exercise can have you lying in bed, completely helpless, for twenty years, or until you die.*

Just to back this up, here are some quotes from some of the most famous doctors who first studied and treated hundreds of patients with this illness:

Sir Donald Acheson, former UK Chief Medical Officer, wrote about ME/CFS:

> *"In the management of the acute phase, absolute rest provides the best outcome."*

> *"The association of premature attempts at rehabilitation with relapse are well described." (8)*

While Dr. Melvin Ramsay (the Consultant in Infectious Diseases who spent his whole career after the 1955 Royal Free Hospital outbreak studying this illness) warns:

> *"...in those patients whose dynamic or conscientious temperament urge them to continue efforts despite profound malaise or in those who, on the false assumption of 'neurosis' have been exhorted to 'snap out of it' and 'take plenty of exercise' the*

condition finally results in a state of constant exhaustion."

"The degree of physical incapacity varies greatly, but the dominant clinical feature of profound fatigue is directly related to the length of time the patient persists in physical effort after its onset; put in another way, those patients who are given a period of enforced rest from the onset have the best prognosis." (1)

Did I mention anything about REST?

ME is counter-intuitive, and it is very countercultural. We find it easy to understand illnesses which gradually progress towards increasing levels of disability and illness up until death. ME is just the opposite: it begins with a serious level of disability, but from that beginning, ME can progress, very slowly, towards improved functioning, or even a significant degree of recovery. Or it may just continue at the same level. Or, most commonly, it may follow a remitting/relapsing course – usually depending on whether the patient has stayed within activity limits or gone over them. Or it can follow a path of deterioration to the point where the patient is bedridden, sensitive to light and noise, and requires help with every basic function. (4) **It seems that there is a window of opportunity at the very beginning** *of the illness, in which complete rest creates the possibility of movement towards recovery, and lack of it is likely to send the patient towards more severe and long-lasting levels of disability. So much for 'fighting'!*

AT THIS POINT I IMAGINE YOU ARE THINKING 'B****Y REST! BRILLIANT, THANKS A LOT FOR THAT! THEN WHAT?'

I hate the concept of spending my life resting, and I expect you do, too. So having told you to rest as much as possible, I will make some suggestions for managing the logistics of an illness which requires you to rest. My suggestions are based on the concept of conserving energy, initially for the basic, completely unavoidable tasks that make up coping with everyday life. If/when you improve enough, you will be trying to work out ways of conserving enough energy to enable you to return to a modified version of your job or domestic (hard!) work. (Ramsay points out the particular difficulty for a woman with children to care for, of getting enough rest to have any chance of recovery. (1)) The critical issue here is that all the while you need to be maintaining sufficient energy reserves so that your body can keep doing whatever it needs to do to keep you on a path towards getting better rather than getting worse.

The conundrum which you need to understand and help those around you to understand arises from the paradoxical nature of ME. You need to adopt the lifestyle of an invalid, a disabled person, *now,* in order to create the possibility of gradually returning towards a more normal future. Failure to do so can result in eventual permanent disability. Which do you want? Which do those around you want for you?

But before going into all that, I want to tell you about Les Simpson's work, because he has done years of research into the relationship of red blood cell functioning and the symptoms of ME. Les knows there are some things you can try which may considerably improve your well-being and give you a head start on that pathway towards recovery.

(If you want to learn about Les's work in more depth, my longer book, 'Common Sense about ME'(forthcoming) includes a chapter based on an article he wrote for Positive Health magazine (9), and 'Ramsay's Disease – ME' (10) incorporates the book he has written about his work. This book also includes a detailed history of the medical and political developments concerning this illness, and his commentary on several commonly used guidelines).

But if this next section looks too technical, skip over it, and come back later on if you want to. The important bit is his recommendations, which are in the section after this one, titled 'And the Good News is?'

HEMORHEOLOGY - EXPLAINING THE SYMPTOMS OF ME

Think about our most basic needs for survival: food, water, and air.

We can live without food for several weeks; without water for just a few days; without air for just a few minutes. Why? Every cell, tissue and organ in our body depends upon our red blood cells absorbing oxygen from the air in our lungs, transporting it throughout our body, removing waste products from our cells, and travelling back to our lungs to discharge carbon dioxide and absorb more oxygen.

Yet hemorheology – the study of the physical properties of blood, including the shape and flexibility (deformability) of our red blood cells – is not taught in medical school. This means that its implications for the treatment of many illnesses are not part of general medical knowledge.

Medical students are taught that all red blood cells are 'biconcave discocytes' – round, flat, with a dimple on each side. This shape is very flexible (deformable) and it is the deformability of the red blood cells which allows them to travel through the smallest of our blood vessels, the capillaries, to carry out their functions. The red blood cells are two to three times wider than the tiny blood vessels they must pass through, so their deformability is essential to the normal functioning of every cell, tissue and organ in our body.

Les's research (10), (11), (12) (13), shows that in many chronic conditions, including ME, the red blood cell population, which is extremely sensitive to changes in its environment, becomes dominated by shape-changed cells. There are at least six cell variations including cup forms, ones with irregular edges, etc. all of which are stiff (non-deformable) and therefore unable to traverse the capillaries.

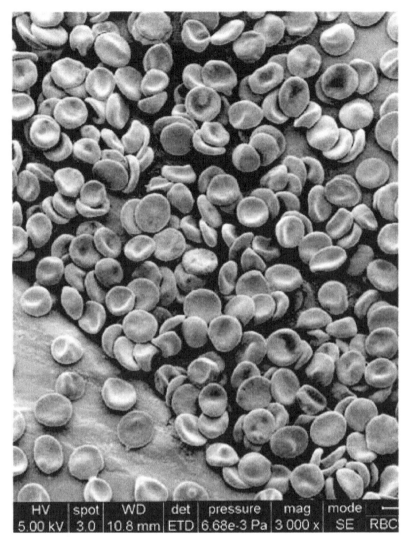

Figure 1 - My Blood Micrograph

'Figure 1 - My Blood Micrograph' is one of a set made from a sample of the author's blood, immediately fixed, on 8th July 2010. The author has had ME since 1986; Dr Les

Simpson's statistical analysis indicated that the shape populations were consistent with chronic ME. The Micrographs were taken by the Experimental Officer, Electron Microscopy Unit, at The School of Pharmacy, University of London.

How many cells do you see in this photo that are round, flat, and have a dimple (the biconcave discocyte shape). How many do you see that are different from that?

It is not surprising, then, that tissues and organs which are particularly sensitive to lack of oxygen and build-up of waste products (oxidative and nitrosative stress) will begin to perform badly. These include the muscles, the cognitive areas of the brain, and the endocrine systems which regulate bodily functions. Suddenly, instead of sounding like the incoherent ravings of a hypochondriac, the range of symptoms which occurs in ME finds an explanation that seems to make sense of it all.

Furthermore, Les's research shows that the variations in patient well-being (the relapsing-remitting pattern) are matched by the variations in the red blood cell shape populations. During periods of remission, the red blood cell population returns to a normal distribution of the biconcave discocyte shapes along with the much smaller proportion of other shapes typical in a healthy person.

Research purporting to show that these shape changes are either unimportant or non-existent will be found to rely on a standard way of processing blood samples before taking micrographs. This involves washing the cells in saline and leaving a time delay, during which the red blood cells which have altered shapes will revert to the biconcave discocyte form, supporting the (erroneous) medical dogma that all red blood cells always have this shape.

Les learned that when the blood samples were 'immediately fixed', a procedure used when blood samples are studied during surgery, the shape changes remain apparent, and he always uses this technique with his samples.

Les points out that his research does not explain the cause or causes of ME, which remain unknown. *What it does explain is the mechanism by which the symptoms are produced.*

AND THE GOOD NEWS IS?

The good news for us, for people who have ME, is that there are several relatively easily available supplements which can improve blood flow, and improved blood flow will mean that our symptoms are lessened.

Confusingly, one thing which improves blood flow is gentle exercise. This is what Les has to say about this:

> *"It is important that ME people have some degree of activity, the level of which is determined by the patient. During rest periods, energy stores are replenished to a level consistent with the level of blood flow impairment. Over-activity results in severe depletion of energy stores in muscles as well as adding to blood flow problems which will delay energy replenishment. This is why a treatment aimed at improving blood flow is important."* (14)

(Note that for a person with acute ME, the stage of 'over-activity', represented by the shift from the aerobic to the anaerobic muscle metabolism, can be reached after even very slight exertion - or no exertion at all, if the patient is already suffering from post-exertional malaise. (15), (16))

For purposes of improving blood flow, Les has found that 4g per day of genuine Evening Primrose Oil may make a significant improvement in our well-being, by improving the flexibility of the red blood cells. He emphasizes the importance of this amount, even though it will be twice the recommendation you will see on the container. (His research has also exposed the fact that only a few products which describe themselves as EPO are in fact genuine, so you need to be sure of your source.)

If a six-week trial of EPO taken at the level Les recommends does not have any noticeable effect, then he would suggest trying 6g per day of fish oil. (Fish oil is recommended for a number of other conditions, so taking it is probably a good idea regardless of effect on ME.) Again he would emphasize the importance of taking the amount he recommends, and he would again suggest a six week trial to find out for yourself whether it is going to help you.

His two further suggestions are Vitamin B12, given as hydroxocobalamin, and pentoxifylline. You would probably need a doctor's prescription for either of these. It may be helpful if your doctor is aware that that Vitamin B12 as hydroxocobalamin has been a fairly traditional treatment for fatigue.

Les would reiterate that these will help only a significant percentage of patients, and that he does not know why they are helpful for some and not for others. (He also doesn't sell any of them, so his recommendations are made only because he wants to help people who have ME.) And he does not claim that they will 'cure' ME – only that they may improve your well-being. You can start your own trial!

BACK TO THINGS YOU CAN DO TO SAVE ENERGY

Most people with ME figure these strategies out for themselves. The main problem lies in convincing yourself and others that *these energy-conserving measures,* however trivial or silly (or over-the-top) they may sound *are as necessary to your getting better as any form of medication could be for any serious illness.*

It is difficult to make many general recommendations because so much depends on the type of house you live in (do you have a lavatory on each floor?), your family situation (do you live alone or is someone else available to help?; do you have children to take care of?), the nature of your job – how much physical exertion does it require?, can it be adapted to conserve your energy?; your financial circumstances (can you afford to pay for help and/or mechanical aids, such as an intercom?)

Whatever your situation may be, you need to become a time-and-motion study expert on the subject of muscular exertion. This involves applying yourself to minimising use of that very scarce resource! Lie rather than sit, sit rather than stand, ask someone else to do whatever it is rather than doing it yourself. (This is one reason why we people who have ME have such a bad reputation – we really do *have to* become very demanding – but remember that being very appreciative should go along with that. Saying 'Thank you, I'm sorry to have to ask, and I'm really grateful for your help' doesn't take much muscular exertion!)

Now, there is one important issue which is always overlooked. Suppose I asked you to carry an eight-pound bowling ball around with you, all of the time? You would probably think that was a pretty unreasonable request to make, especially of a sick person. But that is precisely what you are doing day in, day out because your head weighs about eight pounds and your neck muscles are doing the carrying. If you make a habit of freeing yourself from that particular expenditure of energy, by making sure that your head is always supported (using a recliner, a high-backed chair or the nearest wall) you will find that it does make a difference. I got a fairly high-powered job soon after I became ill, which involved going to meetings and writing reports, so I could do it in my own time, coming home to rest between each activity. I found that if I could keep my head supported in a meeting, I could keep track of what was going on, but the reverse was also true. If there was no way I could lean against something, I would quickly lose the plot and find myself becoming increasingly unable to follow what was going on. (Sometimes, in desperation, I had to drape myself in some rather undignified postures, or back my chair up against a wall, but it was absolutely essential to do that.) This one tip can make a surprising difference – freeing you from this particular unnecessary exertion in order to be able to do the most essential things (in this example, my being able to keep track of a complicated discussion).

Make shameless use of every labour-saving device you can find. I found it necessary to use a wheelchair – necessary, and very liberating. You need the transit kind, designed to be pushed by someone else. (My dog learned to pull me about, as a variant of the tugging game some dogs love – they get hold of something, you try to get it away from them and, if you happen to be in a wheelchair, you can find yourself flying along! Dogs as disability aids are much more common now, though I don't yet know of ones trained to help people with ME.) But when you are semi-mobile, a wheelchair can double-up as something to lean on as you are walking along (put your parcels, or your suitcase, in the wheelchair, and use your weight, rather than your muscles, to propel it forward), a seat to sit in when you get tired - or a modified fair ride if you are with a playful companion! Just because you have a wheelchair doesn't mean you have to sit in it all the time - or be boring! (Admittedly, bystanders do get a little sceptical when you get up out of a wheelchair, especially if you then go up some stairs – but that's their problem, not yours. Remember that. Try not to waste energy worrying what other people may think – they are not the ones who will be in bed for a week if you try to save their embarrassment by doing something that is beyond what your illness allows you.)

And this reminds me of advice given by Dr. Betty Dowsett (17): save your energy to do just a little of the things you enjoy. (I used to go to the local night-club in a wheelchair, and get up for just one very minimalist dance...that confused the onlookers!)

Tasks have to be divided up and done a bit at a time, with rests in between. If you have to iron (and can do it at all, it's not really good to be lifting the weight of an iron repeatedly) at least get a stool so you can sit while you do it. If you live in a two-story house – let's hope you have an upstairs and a downstairs loo, because going upstairs is very tiring. Don't carry your heavy electric kettle to the sink but instead carry water (only as much as you need) in a light plastic jug to the kettle. Deal with doors that stick and furniture that needs moving (a really bad thing to do!) with the weight of your backside and not with the muscles of your arms. In fact, there are lots of situations in which the use of your body-weight can substitute for the use of muscle power.

You want to remain a part of your family, but you need to lie down, a lot. I found one of those garden recliners, with a panel for your legs, in which you can change the angle just by lifting the arms and making a simple movement, really useful, if you can overcome objections to having one in the house. A recliner allows you (easily and fairly unobtrusively) to move from lying down to sitting up, and offers various options in between, to accommodate what you are doing (reading, watching TV, talking on the phone, chatting with a friend, using a laptop, or sleeping). You can rest at a moment's notice, for as little or as long as you need to, without even the bother of moving from lying down to sitting up on a settee. You are an invalid, having to rest just about all of the time. But you don't need to do it in bed or in isolation from your family and friends. Your invalid status can be relatively disguised – *not by making heroic efforts to behave normally when you know that makes you worse* – but simply by having the right piece of furniture. And of course, recliners come in all styles and price ranges – it's just that the garden ones are very inexpensive and uncomplicated.

At this point I feel as though I should be offering prizes for further tips on muscle economy! You know what you have to do and you know your own situation better than anyone else. You can be creative in thinking up more ways to be 'energy efficient' with your own body, both in how you do (and don't do) the things you have to do, and in adapting your environment as much as you can, and getting the right equipment . (If anyone dares to criticise, just tell them that as soon as they have experienced ME themselves, their advice will be very welcome.)

By now you will have noticed that although I am warning you that you have a serious illness – which by all reports goes on for a long time, and will definitely be made worse by exertion – and I am even telling you to adopt the lifestyle of an invalid, a disabled person – it isn't about spending all your time in bed being miserable and lonely. It is about how to slot that energy-conserving lifestyle into a life that appears as normal as possible. This approach involves saving energy in order to construct a semblance of normal living as well as getting your working circumstances adapted so that you can go on leading the life of an employed person, if at all possible. It is about saving the energy your body needs so that you can gradually improve, while still managing a range of your normal activities. The more ruthless you are about conserving energy, the more you will be able to do.

I did say that this illness is paradoxical!

AND WHAT ABOUT THE PSYCHOLOGICAL FACTORS?
(NO, *NOT* THE ONES THE PSYCHIATRISTS GO ON ABOUT!)

Right now, you are sick. But you know, and I know *who you are*, beyond this illness. You are energetic, conscientious and ambitious. You always go the extra mile. You have high standards for yourself in everything you do. When you get sick, which isn't very often, you still do all you can to meet your commitments. You have interests that you are excited about; you enjoy your family and friends. If you have been criticized in the past, the 'criticisms' are most likely to have been expressions of concern – that you do too much, you put others first, you don't take care of yourself - never that you are lazy, or don't pull your weight.

Maybe, if this illness has crept up gradually, you have had some spells when you couldn't live up to your own expectations; you got sick and didn't seem to be able to pull out of it. Then, after a few weeks, you were OK again, and you carried on. This is pretty much what happened to me, before the final time when I got this weird kind of flu, and just didn't get better. And maybe that's how it is for you now.

Maybe you have been travelling abroad, and seem to have 'picked up something'. (It's quite likely that your travel was the back-packing kind – adventurous, physically demanding.)

Maybe you have always enjoyed strenuous sports, and are a high achiever in whichever sports you engage in. You are likely to have been, at the very least, the sort of person who is conscientious about work-outs, jogging and keeping fit.

So when this illness comes out of the blue, *it is totally alien to the kind of person that you are.* When you find yourself just going limp, for no obvious reason, and it goes on and goes on, you feel more than just sick. You are losing not just the activities you used to do - you may be threatened about losing your job, your income, with all that that would mean, or you find yourself unable to take proper care of your children. Your family or partner may even be sceptical and unhelpful, believing it is best to tell you to 'pull yourself together'. (You only wish you could!) And if they are sympathetic and helpful, you feel terribly guilty about being a burden, more so because there is no visible reason for your being so incapacitated.

But, even more disturbingly, this illness forces you to change your way of living to such a degree that you may even feel you are losing your sense of your identity – the person you have always believed yourself to be, the person you want to continue to be. That is the most profound psychological challenge of all.

And in the face of all that, I come along and tell you to stop fighting, lie down and accept living like a very sick, very disabled person. How can you possibly do that and retain any self-respect? That must sound to you like the worst possible advice – a complete violation of who you are.

Yet you have to, right now, if you want to have any hope of ultimate recovery.

You need the help of a mentor, a counsellor or a psychotherapist who will support you in the knowledge that what you are suffering from is an illness with a complex physiological basis. (You need someone who is not just saying these words to avoid upsetting you, but rather, because they actually know them to be true). You need the help and support of such a person in giving yourself permission to take the rest you need – not to give in and be a victim - but because it is simply the only way to get better. You need help to let go of your own self-criticism, your inappropriate guilt for being this sick and your underlying conviction that you ought to be engaged in the effort to do more.

That is what you *need*. What you will *get*, from the medical establishment in the UK, and many other countries, is the injustice of being labelled along with 'hypochondriacs' (people who are terrified that they have an illness, but they don't) and 'malingerers' (people who deliberately pretend to have an illness in order to get attention/sympathy/incapacity benefits) as a person with a 'somatoform disorder': a psychiatric category. The psychiatrists insist that this illness results from people (often after having a viral illness) paying too much attention to normal physical sensations, exaggerating them and, as a result, getting very anxious about them. According to the psychiatric view it is anxiety that causes people to adopt an invalid lifestyle: a lifestyle which avoids exertion and causes 'deconditioning'. The cure (the psychiatrists say that CFS is 'completely reversible') is to use Cognitive Behaviour Therapy. This therapy is designed to convince you that it is your thinking which is at fault, and then to persuade (or coerce) you into doing Graded Exercise Therapy. GET, they assure us, will get you over your 'deconditioning', improve your physical fitness, and help you to regain normal muscular strength. (18) (But in a study by Bazelmans et al, 'There were no statistically significant differences in physical fitness between CFS patients and their controls.' (19))

They will tell you that there has been a big research trial which has shown that CBT and GET are helpful in this illness. (20) (And they will tell your doctor to assure you that he believes your illness is 'real', because it is OK to say something to patients which they will take to mean one thing, while the doctor actually means something completely different. (21))

This group of psychiatrists accuse ME/CFS patients of 'scenting the possibility of a career'. Actually, a career as an ME patient is neither lucrative nor rewarding. However, the career of a psychiatrist making his living on the backs of very physically sick people must be, judging by the enormous amount of effort that has gone into categorising ME/CFS as a psychiatric illness. Their aim is to label ME as a 'chronic somatoform symptom disorder' in the latest edition of the Diagnostic and Statistical Manual of Psychiatric Disorders (DSM- V).

(While we are on the subject of diagnoses, there is some interesting research on the organisational 'sociopath'. (22) (23))

My final footnote on all of the above is that the psychiatrists are doing a great disservice to malingerers and hypochondriacs by lumping them together with ME/CFS sufferers. *No hypochondriac would (or could!) make up the wildly diverse and improbable set of symptoms which characterise ME. Even if they were that creative, it's obvious that no one would believe them. And no malingerer worth his salt would waste his time feigning an illness which generates so much contempt and disbelief.*

SO WHAT <u>SHOULD</u> THE DOCTORS BE DOING?

"Do No Harm"

The Hippocratic Oath

The first thing they should do (and the International Consensus Criteria (4) confirm this) is give you an interim diagnosis straight away, so that you can start resting while they do the routine tests to eliminate other possible causes of your symptoms.

During the discussion at the end of the Invest in ME June Conference (2012), a doctor said 'We take our patients into hospital while we do the assessments. And my patients get better.' (24) This should be standard medical procedure, but only *if a hospital stay will provide the enforced rest which Ramsay recommends*. (There is a serious danger, especially if you are hospitalised as a psychiatric admission, of treatment based on the idea that a combination of bullying and neglect can force you into the desired level of activity, to demonstrate that you are not really ill. (25))

ME/CFS needs to be treated as the serious illness that it is. Given the very stark choices which it presents (either progress towards recovery, or progress towards very severe and long-lasting or permanent disabling illness) **the prescription for rest needs to be taken as seriously as one would take the prescription of any drug or medical procedure for a comparable illness**. (But neither the drug companies nor the psychiatrists stand to profit from this prescription, so it is very unlikely to be forthcoming.)

Apart from Les' recommendations for supplements which can improve well-being considerably in a reasonable percentage of patients, and the prescription of Rituximab (26), which is still in the experimental stage, we do not have a treatment for ME. (There are a number of other drugs, such as Ampligen, being trialled, but it can be prohibitively expensive just to join a trial, as participants can be expected to pay for their own, very costly, drugs.) Many people who have ME use a range of supplements, some of which are helpful. But the bottom line is that what we have is what we had for TB years ago, before the development of antibiotics. As with TB in those days, people who have ME are reliant on the body's own resources for dealing with whatever constitutes the agent or dysfunction that is causing this illness. Even when we do finally have effective drugs, and it is looking more and more likely that we will have, perhaps within the next few years, they will be expensive and not available to everyone, or at least, not for a long time. *Our best hope is for the body to be given the chance to direct all its energies and resources towards dealing with this complex, multi-system problem that affects us.*

This means that people with ME need to be treated with respect: their descriptions of their symptoms, and their accounts of how things affect them should be assumed to be both truthful and accurate, and responded to accordingly.

We are not lazy. We do want to get better. We are not imagining or exaggerating our situations. We are not suffering from depression, or lack of motivation. We lie down because we have to, not because we are fans of lying down. We are terribly frustrated at our inability to continue our jobs, our education, our schooling, if we are children, we miss playing with our friends.

(Children who avoid school for psychological reasons come home and go out to play – children who have ME, when they can go to school at all, come home and go to bed.) We do not find any advantages in being sick. We do not want to be waited on: we want to be able to do things for ourselves, and for others. It is time that we were

respected, and allowed to do what we need to do to get better. We should not be forced into treatments which involve lying to us, insulting our intelligence and our integrity, and which can ultimately deprive us of our chance to recover.

So, our message to the doctors is as follows: Support us in our need for complete rest at the beginning; support us in our continuing need to be ruthless in our attempts to conserve energy so that we can manage a semblance of our ordinary life. Support us in rationing our activities to enable our bodies achieve some degree of recovery. And, please, support us in dealing with the blood flow issues – trying out each of Les Simpson's suggestions until we find the one that works best for us.

AND THE MESSAGE FOR PUBLIC POLICY?

In my constant study of the latest research developments, I have become aware of a trend towards describing ME as an illness which tends to get worse, and some researchers are even wondering whether it is a naturally 'progressive' illness. This is in sharp contrast to those early researchers who noted that patients who had complete rest during the early stages tended to recover.

I am convinced that this trend is nothing to do with the nature of ME as an illness – it is an outcome of the fact that so many of us are enduring treatments and treatment approaches which are known to make us worse. This should be of major concern to the Department of Health and the Department of Work and Pensions.

In the days of Ramsay and Acheson, hospital treatment implied enforced bed rest, and their patients did get better. Today a hospital admission risks both brutality and neglect by staff who are encouraged to believe that these sick people are 'just trying it on', and that it is even acceptable to refuse extremely sick patients any help at all, in order to force them into activity. (See, for example, the case of Sophia Mirza, on the ME Action website. (25))

With Norway taking the lead (13), our public and medical authorities need to take a very firm line in following the International Consensus Criteria for ME, and, in so doing, remove this illness (however named) firmly out of the remit of the psychiatric profession.

Like many previous illnesses (for example, MS, epilepsy, duodenal ulcers to name but a few) ME/CFS has provided fodder for the psychiatric profession because its physiological nature has not been understood. A misdiagnosed headache that signals a tumour, the heart condition treated as a panic attack, the insidious progress of thyroid problems treated with antidepressants: mistaken psychiatric diagnoses can have fatal consequences.

Regarding ME/CFS in light of the above claim, we know that early treatment will determine either progress towards recovery or permanent disability. And yet, the psychiatric dogma that says you must tell the patient that their symptoms are just 'false illness beliefs', and that their reluctance to exercise must be firmly discouraged means that *treatment based on the idea that ME is a 'somatoform disorder' is pretty well guaranteed to push patients towards permanent disability.* This situation really must not be allowed to continue.

As long as taxpayers are funding payments to people who are ill or disabled, the Government will want to get people back to work as quickly as possible. ***But it does not make economic sense to force sick people into activities which will prolong their illness and make their disability worse. This is especially the case when a completely different approach could increase the probability of a return to normal or nearly normal health.***

The psychiatrists and the rehabilitation experts have persuaded the government, the media and the health community that their approach works. A close analysis of the research that is used to justify such belief (27) (28), (29), along with an extension of the sources of information that are available to include the wide range of research proving that this illness is not a psychiatric complaint would allow us to reach a very different conclusion.

But if medical research is not read, if reviews are confined to papers written by psychiatrists, if conferences on the medical aspects of CFS/ME are not reported, if a search of the Royal Society of Medicine library of medical journals does not come up with even one reference to the hundreds of research papers on CFS or ME which have appeared in their journals, we will continue to go round in the same narrow circles.

In the current atmosphere, which celebrates disabled athletes on the one hand, and wages a campaign to label the disabled as welfare scroungers on the other, people who have ME are increasingly disadvantaged. Told that we are just exaggerating minor complaints, and that we should 'get over it', we can't display any athletic heroism to prove that we are really good guys, fighting our disability. We are the absolute opposite of anything that our culture admires. 'Complainers', 'lazy', 'giving up'....and no one hates those qualities more than we do! You would have to have known us before we were sick, to know that we are not those people. We do not choose this illness. But try to sell that to the media....

AND, REALLY IMPORTANT: FOR OUR CARERS

If you have read all of this, you will already have a lot of good ideas about what your patient with ME needs from you (a lot!). It won't make you instantly happy, but may be helpful for you to remind yourself that every time you do something that rescues your patient from having to use their muscles, you are making a positive contribution towards the possibility of their improvement. You've been doing all the work, to a ridiculous extent, for a long time, and I would guess having to struggle against feeling put upon, resentful and used. It is likely that you've been feeling helpless in the face of this illness that goes on and on and on. In fact, you may be feeling completely and utterly fed up with the situation. And the temptation is never far away – family members, friends and complete strangers will be saying it to you as well – to think that if only your patient would keep trying to do a bit more, it would be bound to make them feel better. It is difficult to avoid the thought that they should be fighting against their illness and trying harder. They want to believe this, too! Yet whenever they do make that extra effort they inevitably get worse, sometimes much worse.

Can you begin to believe what those early experts (not today's psychiatrists!) had to say? Complete rest *is* what your patient needs to get better, even though resting doesn't seem to make much immediate difference. If you can accept this as fact then you might begin to know, to feel in your bones, that *every time you do something that saves your patient using their muscles, you are making a positive contribution to their ultimate progress. This is the truth of the matter – the most important role you can perform.*

If your patient were actually paralyzed, it would be completely clear that it was necessary to help in this way. The person with ME is in a very similar situation, but the similarity isn't clear-cut enough to be beyond question by those who want to question it. We intuitively 'know' that when muscles are used they get stronger. When muscles are not used they get weaker. Except that this 'knowledge' doesn't apply to ME sufferers. It really doesn't.

If you've been watching the Olympics, you will have seen athletes performing at the very limit of their strength and capacity: witness the tearful collapse at the end of the marathon, the swimming, the boxing match or the weight-lifting. No-one would dream of suggesting to these athletes that what they needed to do was more of the same, that immediately running another race, or lifting another weight, would be good for them. You know that if they were pushed beyond their limits, something would give and some damage would be done. Their coaches will be taking care of them by making sure they let their muscles have a chance to recover.

Your patient reaches that point after the slightest effort because of a failure in the normal muscle metabolism. They are already in that state. The nature of ME is such that *they are at the end of their marathon, all day every day.* If you can understand that then maybe you can become the coach who is determined to protect your athlete from the damage that is done when anything further is asked of them.

This protective mind-set may help you to understand what is needed and the importance and value of your contribution. When you feel as though you are just doing one unrewarding and endless chore after another, remind yourself that every chore you do is helping to create the possibility for your athlete to recover. There are no medical cures, as yet, supplements to improve blood flow will often produce marked improvement – but your ongoing efforts are the best medicine of all.

KEEP UP THE GOOD FIGHT BY REFUSING TO FIGHT!

Our very best wishes, and hopes for your progress towards recovery; we hope we've been helpful!

BY THE WAY, WHO ARE NANCY BLAKE AND LES SIMPSON?

Nancy is a retired social worker and a very experienced psychotherapist, who became ill with ME in 1986. She knows that ME is a physical illness, not a psychological condition, and she knows that in order to get better we have to accept that the way to fight ME is to rest as much as possible. The only way forward is by saving our energy to do the basics, and a little bit of what we enjoy, leaving enough energy over for our bodies to gradually recover.

Les has studied problems of blood flow for more than thirty years, and he spent six years going all over the world while continuing his research into ME, attending scientific meetings, conferences and ME support groups, including visiting severely ill patients in their home.

He explains that our symptoms are caused by stiffened red blood cells that can't deliver oxygen properly to our muscles and brain. Taking Genuine Evening Primrose Oil or fish oil can improve our blood flow, and many of us will experience significant improvement from following these suggestions.

You are very welcome to write to either of us, at the addresses below:

Nancy Blake, alternatives@alternatives.karoo.co.uk

Les Simpson, leslie.simpson@slingshot.co.nz

Summary

Is your illness ME?

You've been busy, active, ambitious, conscientious, helpful, and enjoying life, but now…

You can hardly move, you are very, very tired for days after minimal exertion and you have trouble thinking and remembering, plus many other apparently random symptoms. These symptoms include headaches, sore throat, swollen glands, painful muscles and they all vary from day to day, even hour to hour. You really don't understand it. You may have ME.

Rest is the most immediate and essential treatment.

If you have ME, the most important thing to do is to rest – immediately. In the past, those people who were taken care of in hospital, right from the beginning, were the ones who recovered, or at least improved. (But remember, that was when people with ME in hospital were allowed to rest.)

People who 'fight it' get worse, sometimes terribly worse, for a long time. The motto for anyone who has ME should be *GIVE IN, TO GET WELL.*

Ask your doctor to run diagnostic tests to eliminate anything else.

Get your doctor to give you a normal set of diagnostic tests to rule out anything else that might be causing it. If everything appears normal then that can be considered as 'diagnosis by elimination': confirmation that you have ME.

Take genuine EPO, or fish oil.

In the course of thirty years of research into ME, Les Simpson has found that taking 4g of genuine Evening Primrose Oil or 6 g of fish oil every day has helped a lot of people with ME. Improvement can occur because stiffened red blood cells can be stopping oxygen getting to your muscles and your brain and, in many cases, these supplements can help. It is worth trying. If these do not help, see if you can persuade your doctor to prescribe Vitamin B12 as hydroxocobalamin, or pentoxyfilline.

Avoid CBT and GET if at all possible.

Try to avoid getting any treatment involving cognitive behaviour therapy (to persuade you that you don't have a physical illness – you do) and graded exercise therapy (to help you recover from your 'deconditioning' – your muscles aren't 'deconditioned' (19)). You will find out, they will tell you, that you can build strength through exercise (you can't because your muscle metabolism is not working normally. (30). Unfortunately, most 'specialist' units for ME/CFS in this country will be staffed by psychologists, psychiatrists, or occupational therapists who believe in these treatments. (However, there are places, and individual staff, who understand your illness, and whose care may be genuinely helpful. If their version of CBT is to help you adapt to your situation, and their version of GET is to let you be in complete control of what you do, and take care to avoid over-exertion, you have a better chance of benefitting from their involvement or at least not being harmed by it.)

But you may have to be polite about what is on offer, if disability help depends on it.

According to the NICE Guidelines, refusing a particular treatment should not be held against you in any way. Practically speaking, you may be refused any disability payments unless you cooperate with some treatment regime. If this is the case, you have no choice except to smile sweetly and do your best to simulate cooperation while continuing to conserve your energy as much as possible.

Get professional advocacy help if you need to claim benefits.

If you need to claim any sort of financial help on the basis of disability, seek out the help and advice of someone who has experience working as an advocate for people in this situation. Recent government policies are making such claims even more difficult for us. The ME Association website offers advice. There are also useful guidelines on filling out the new Employment Support Allowance forms at www.nawra.org.uk, (31) and advice specifically for people with ME at www.shropshiremegroup.org.uk (32)

Become a time-and-motion expert in saving physical energy

You will find that the need to minimise physical (and mental) exercise continues for a long time. Do your best to organise your life (and your furniture!) so that everything is as physically easy as possible.

Be really grateful to your carers – this isn't their fault!

You cannot manage without a lot of physical help. But you've always been the one who helped others and you hate being helpless. Also you feel terribly guilty about needing all this care and assistance. (This guilt is why a lot of invalids get peevish and horrible. Don't get peevish and horrible.) Right now, you do need it, so do your best to let go of the guilt and just make sure that you let your helpers know that you are grateful for what they do.

Carers – you are actively helping this person have a chance to get better!

Anyone who is helping you or caring for you needs to know that every bit of exertion they save you from is a bit of energy your body can use to work toward your recovery. The endless round of tedious, trivial physical tasks that they do for you is the best medicine you can have, the best possible gift they can give you.

Finally, if anyone tells you it's all in your head and you should just snap out of it, tell them to come back to you on that one when they've got ME themselves. (And in the meantime, just snap out of your life! You really don't need that kind of 'advice'.)

LIST OF HELPFUL WEBSITES

National Alliance for Myalgic Encephalomyelitis www.name-us.org includes definitions and articles from the earliest researchers – Ramsay, Acheson, and Dowsett.

One Click - www.theoneclickgroup.co.uk Put ME/CFS into their search engine to find an article 'Mobilising ME/CFS Charities to Smash Flawed PACE Trial Results, by Lara Hessler, 14/4/2011. This explains the changes to the disability assessment system as of that time (there are further changes taking place at the moment – August 2012). Her suggestion is that ME Charities should pay for individual patients to have medical tests (not allowed by the NICE Guidelines) to prove that they are not suffering from ME/CFS as defined by PACE, but have a biologically-based condition.

You can access the full text of the Myalgic Encephalomyelitis: International Consensus Criteria by putting this into their search line and clicking onto the

Google reference, which will bring up a page on it, go to the bottom of the page and click onto 'Full Text'.

For a very scientific explanation of why CBT and GET are harmful, go onto One Click, and type in 'Twisk and Maes'.

Invest in ME, www.investinme.org provides reports on research and on their annual conferences. This is the source of the information about development in Norway – the Rituximab trials, in which some patients have been cured. (26) These have resulted in a government apology to people with ME/CFS who have been told their illness was a 'behavioural' problem, and treated with CBT and GET. They now recommend against these treatments. (13)

ME-CFS Community, at www.me-cfscommunity.com or www.cfsknowledgecenter.ning.com will take you to a very helpful site for the most recent research.

IACFSME www.iacfsme.org is a U.S. based site, which is announcing the formation of a new journal, also they take a definite stand against the proposal to label ME a psychiatric problem in DSM V.

Keeping up with the politics:

MEActionUK, at www.meactionuk.org.uk or on Facebook, www.facebook.com/pages/MEActionUK/287426748781

Help filling out Employment Support Allowance Form

www.nawra.org.uk - Fit For Purpose?

www.shropshiremegroup.org.uk - Hints for Completing the ESA 50 form.

ADDENDA

I think of The Beginner's Guide to ME/CFS as an emergency manual for people who are just discovering that they have ME (or whatever name it is given by the doctor who provides the diagnosis). The Guide is intended to be a brief and simple booklet that even a very ill person can make sense of and benefit from.

'Ramsay's Disease - Myalgic Encephalomyelitis (ME), and the Unfortunate Creation of CFS' (10) is a lengthier book which gives a comprehensive account of the history of ME, including the history of Les Simpson's involvement with ME research, conferences, and patient groups. It also provides detailed information about the science behind Les's recommendations and much more of my story!

Based on the premise that people who have ME/CFS, and their carers may want to go more deeply into different aspects of this illness I am planning to produce further small Beginner's Guides. Future publications will cover the medical research, the political history, the different treatment approaches and the ongoing controversy between the psychiatrists and the rest of us!

In the interests of keeping matters short and simple, I decided not to include some brief Addenda on these issues in the Kindle version of A Beginner's Guide to ME/CFS. However, it seems appropriate to include them here, as indications of material which will be covered more fully in separate 'Beginner's Guides'.

The addition of this section, at the time of going into print, has allowed me to include some information that has appeared since the Kindle edition was produced.

THE ME/CFS NAME GAME

"...inflammation occurs in the brain and there's evidence that patients with this illness experience a level of disability that's equal to that of patients with late-stage AIDS, patients undergoing chemotherapy, or patients with multiple sclerosis."

Dr. Nancy Klimas

"Myalgic encephalomyelitis (ME) is a severe, complex neurological disease that affects all body systems. ME is more debilitating than most diseases." *2012 ICC Physician's Primer*

"We consider [ME/CFS] to be in the category of serious or life threatening diseases."

U.S. Food and Drug Administration

(Quotations from the home page of the National Association for ME, www.name-us.org (33))

The naming of this illness has a long and complicated history which is detailed in 'Ramsay's Disease – Myalgic Encephalomyelitis'. The title of this book signifies Les

Simpson's commitment to the use of Ramsay's original diagnostic criteria. It also testifies to his aim to separate the illness so designated from the confusion caused by the introduction of a wider range of criteria along with the term 'Chronic Fatigue Syndrome'

In the 1950's, Ramsay, and doctors dealing with outbreaks similar to the Royal Free Hospital epidemic which Ramsay studied, eventually settled on the term 'benign myalgic encephalomyelitis' for this illness. In the context of the annual polio epidemics which were causing permanent crippling, and often, death to sufferers, people with ME, who would be admitted to hospital with very similar symptoms, but then recover without permanent paralysis, were considered the lucky ones, hence the term 'benign'. Given the serious and long term illness suffered by people who have ME, this adjective was subsequently dropped.

However, in the context of the polio epidemics, these patients might have been regarded as having been admitted to hospital under false pretences. Perhaps this is one historical factor underlying the hostility to ME patients which appears still to be embedded in our culture.

Years after the 1955 Royal Free Epidemic, Ramsay allowed two psychiatrists, McEvedy and Beard, access to the hospital records of the patients he had treated during the epidemic. These men had apparently focused on the notes of a group of patients whom Ramsay himself had dismissed from his studies as possibly having psychiatric problems. This did not prevent the two psychiatrists from subsequently writing an article which purported to prove that the whole epidemic was an outbreak of 'mass hysteria'. (34) This view was enthusiastically adopted by the medical profession and the media, and has contaminated attitudes towards people with ME ever since.

Since then the development of diagnostic criteria has been a struggle between those who attempt to narrow the diagnosed group to those who have ME, and those who have introduced broader criteria, which allow the inclusion of people with psychiatric and other problems in the diagnosed group. These broader criteria include the Fukuda, used by the US Centre for Disease Control, Reeves, as mentioned below, and the Oxford criteria. (The ME Association website, among others, provides information about these different diagnostic lists.) The label given to the condition that results from these diagnostic criteria is Chronic Fatigue Syndrome, or CFS. To add to the confusion, the labels ME/CFS, or CFS/ME are often bracketed as an extension of the Chronic Fatigue Syndrome label. We also have Fibromyalgia (FM), for people whose illness seems similar but whose main symptom is pain, and Chronic Fatigue Immune Deficiency syndrome (CFIDS), acknowledging that this illness is associated with problems in the immune system.

Generally speaking, the inclusion of broader criteria and the label 'Chronic Fatigue Syndrome' seem to be used for the purpose of maintaining the concept of the illness as a psychiatric problem. People who recognise the physical nature of this illness continue to insist on using the name Myalgic Encephalomyelitis (ME), which is listed in the ICD, the WHO classification of diseases, as a neurological disorder.

The International Consensus Criteria Primer for Medical Practitioners (2012 ICC Physician's Primer, quoted above) describes the current situation:

> *'The label 'chronic fatigue syndrome' (CFS), coined in the 1980s, has persisted due to lack of knowledge of its etiologic agents and pathophysiology. Misperceptions have arisen because the name 'CFS' and its hybrids ME/CFS, CFS/ME and CFS/CF have been used for widely diverse conditions. Patient sets can include those who are seriously ill with ME, many bedridden and unable to care for themselves, to those who have general fatigue or, under the*

Reeves criteria, patients are not required to have any physical symptoms. There is a poignant need to untangle the web of confusion caused by mixing diverse and often overly inclusive patient populations in one heterogeneous, multi-rubric pot called 'chronic fatigue syndrome'. We believe this is the foremost cause of diluted and inconsistent research findings, which hinders progress, fosters scepticism, and wastes limited research monies.'

The intensity of feeling surrounding this confusion is caused by the fact that if this illness is labelled as a psychiatric problem then treatment by CBT and GET can be justified. But if we take Acheson's statements very seriously, as we should, we know that 'complete rest' from the beginning of the illness, gives the best ultimate outcome. And further, it is 'well recorded' that relapse results from 'premature attempts at rehabilitation'. 'Relapse' can be anything from a long-lasting deterioration in ones condition to, as in the case of Sophia Mirza, a relentless downward spiral ending in death. www.sophiaandme.org.uk

The name-game is a game with very high stakes for all concerned.

Given in the form of a list, the symptoms of this illness sound like a random, ridiculously diverse set of complaints.

The result is that they are easy to dismiss, especially when you add the fact that they vary, not just from day to day, but from hour to hour – and they can potentially go on for months and years. This provides a lot of support to anyone who wants to claim the illness is a form of hypochondria, a mental health problem.

Set against this claim is the fact that this same, complex and highly variable set of symptoms has been consistently reported from a number of geographically and historically separate parts of the world, over many years. Is this not too much of a coincidence? How likely is it that people who have never heard of the illness and know nothing about it, can by chance, come up with anything this complicated? The symptom pattern is very recognisable, even to people who 'don't believe in ME'.

ME is often, or perhaps always, preceded by a viral infection. The immune system responds. There is much evidence that in ME, the immune system over-responds, and that ME is an autoimmune disorder.

Hemorheology tells us that red blood cells are extremely sensitive to changes in their environment. Both an original viral infection and the immune system response might be the change in environment which stimulates the shape changes in the red blood cell population shown in ME patients.

The oxygen deprivation caused by the increase in non-deformable red blood cells seems to provide an explanation for the fact that muscle metabolism, the cognitive areas of the brain, and the endocrine system are all affected. Poor oxygen delivery to muscles results in exhaustion after little effort, muscular pain, and delayed and protracted recovery from exertion. Poor oxygen delivery to the cognitive areas of the brain results in confusion, short-term memory problems, 'brain fog'. Poor oxygen delivery to the endocrine system results in dysregulation of biorhythms – disruption in sleep patterns, body temperature regulation, and appetite.

Sore throats, headaches, swollen and painful lymph glands, running a fever, are all indicators of immune system activation.

Marrying the consequences of the blood flow problems and the immune system response, we have a coherent physiological explanation for the otherwise random-seeming collection of symptoms. These are not just products of the patients' imagination!

A DEFINING FEATURE OF ME

The Canadian Guidelines, the International Consensus Criteria and Ramsay's original definition cite the defining feature of ME as a delayed and protracted recovery period following exertion. Ramsay describes this condition as 'neurological disturbance – an unpredictable state of central nervous system exhaustion following mental or physical exertion which may be delayed and require several days for recovery'. (Quoted from NAME-us.org) The International Consensus Criteria, written more than twenty five years later, describes the same phenomenon - now labelling it PENE, Post-Exertional Neuro-Immune Exhaustion.

Any list which *makes this the defining criteria* will be selecting people who do have ME.

Any list which *includes this as one symptom among many, but does not require it for a diagnosis* will select people, some of whom may have ME and some of whom may not.

Any list which *excludes people with this symptom* will choose a group of patients who definitely do not have ME.

Any list which purports to diagnose depression, but *includes symptoms which are actually physical symptoms of ME* will misdiagnose people who have ME as having depression. The Beck Inventory, the Zung Self-Rating Depression Scale, and the Malaise Inventory all include physical symptoms of ME.

(The Malaise Inventory adds another layer of confusion. The delayed exhaustion experienced by people who have ME is often called 'post-exertional malaise'. But the Malaise Inventory is described as a tool for diagnosing depression.)

The purported difficulty in making a differential diagnosis between depression and ME seems to have been created by the way that these questionnaires have been designed. One is tempted to wonder whether that confusion is intentional.

Let me ask you, the reader, whether you would, in a relatively short conversation, be able to tell the difference between someone who felt too apathetic or sad to want to do anything, and someone who was desperate to do things and very upset when they tried and found they couldn't? That is how hard it is to tell the difference between someone who is depressed and someone who has ME.

The allegation that the confusion around the labelling of this illness is a deliberate strategy to mislead the medical profession, the media and the public has been put forward by Anglia ME Action in a paper entitled 'A Call for a Parliamentary Select Committee of Inquiry into UK ME & CFS Policy' (www.angliameaction/docs/wessely-misleading). The term 'myalgic encephyalomyelitis' has been used by the World Health Organisation in its classification of this illness as a neurological complaint, and yet Simon Wessely has insisted that 'patients have named their condition'. He claims that the term myalgic encephalomyelitis is 'the lay label' and further suggests that doctors would only use it to avoid offending patients. Wessely is calling for 'constructive labelling', which in his view 'would mean treating chronic fatigue syndrome as a legitimate illness, acknowledging that it may have a viral trigger (as many patients report), while gradually expanding understanding of the condition to incorporate the psychological and social dimensions.' This is said to be part of an overall strategy to maintain and enhance the public conviction that ME is a psychosocial complaint rather than a medical one.

The influence of this approach can be found in many guidelines and sets of advice, in which CFS is acknowledged as a 'real illness' followed by the advice that

CBT and GET are the only 'evidence-based' treatments available.

The people involved in the name-game are on the one hand, broadly the doctors, researchers and patients who know that ME is a physical disorder, with many recorded physiological signs. And on the other hand, the psychiatrists, health insurers and government bodies who are determined that people who have ME should be diagnosed with a 'functional somatoform disorder' – that it to say, with symptoms created and maintained as a mechanism to acquire the 'secondary gains' of being ill. (They seem to believe that a life lived as a very sick person on a pittance could somehow become a desirable alternative to the successful and rewarding professional careers which many patients previously enjoyed!)

The subtext is financial – ME is immediately severely disabling – very expensive for insurers and for agencies funding support for people with disabilities. Once people are given a psychiatric label then the insurers do not have to make disability payments and, from the psychiatrists' point of view, the patients themselves can be blamed when treatment fails. Current UK policies also favour avoiding making disability payments to patients on the grounds that ME/CFS is a psychiatric problem. (See below the reference to Professor Malcolm Hooper's recent letter to Iain Duncan Smith, Secretary of State for Work and Pensions.)

For patients, the immediate consequences can be horrendous – up to and including compulsory admission into a mental health facility. On admission, all forms of physical assistance may be withdrawn, with the intention of forcing the patient to take care of him/her self, which he/she may not be able to do, as in the case of Sophia Mirza.

At or around the time when criticisms of the PACE Trial were beginning to appear in Lancet (28) (29) (35), Simon Wessely (now 'Sir') went onto Radio 4 (36), not to defend PACE, but to complain of having received death threats from ME patients objecting to his views. He claimed this would discourage research into ME, and deplored the unwillingness of ME patients to accept 'the stigma' of a psychiatric diagnosis. He hinted that this, sadly, would deprive such patients of an opportunity to get better. Elsewhere, he has claimed that CFS is 'completely reversible', and that he has been able to help about 30% of his patients. It remains puzzling why such a large cohort of individuals who have been cured of this unpleasant and debilitating illness have not come forward in his defence. And why the promised results of the PACE Trial have not yet been published.

Moving on, let us now consider the ME patient from the point of view of an ethically practicing psychotherapist. In psychotherapy there are diagnostic principles which I believe all practising therapists should take very seriously.

The very first principle is that one must listen very carefully to one's patient's account (and it helps to assume that our patient is telling the truth). Then we have a moral and professional obligation to *recognize the limits of our profession*. If we hear anything that might *signal a medical problem, our first responsibility is to send our client to their doctor to have this symptom investigated.* We do not treat medical problems, although we may be able to help people deal with the emotional impact of medical problems.

Our next diagnostic principle is that we are looking for *a narrative* in the patient's life which might explain why a particular type of problem has arisen. Depression is understandable in the context of a history of bereavements or of relationships in which a person has been physically or emotionally abused. Anxiety is understandable in the context of early separations from important carers, facing a major threat to health or relationships, or to ones employment. Many psychiatric symptoms are preceded by both early traumatic experiences and recently occurring triggers. Whenever there is a relevant narrative, I will expect the client to benefit from psychotherapy.

However, if symptoms arise 'out of the blue' and there doesn't seem to be a narrative that makes sense of it, I will be sending the client back to their doctor for another thorough examination. The history of psychiatric treatment includes the corpses of too many people mistakenly labelled mentally ill, and as a therapist, I do not wish to become part of that history. (For that matter, as a person with ME, I do not wish to become part of that history!)

The narrative of many, many people who suddenly find themselves completely incapacitated by ME is that of someone who is generally exceptionally energetic, ambitious, physically active and enjoying a successful and happy life. In the absence of any history or any trauma that could possibly produce the extreme changes which occur when a person falls ill with ME, I cannot be persuaded that this patient has a psychiatric problem.

However, as the following paragraphs will make clear, it seems that these principles no longer apply.

During the protracted discussions taking place in 2010 and 2011 in the process of revising DSM IV in order to produce the new edition, DSM 5, the psychiatrists were busy setting up a new category 'complex somatoform symptoms disorder' (CSSD). By 2012, this category has become 'SSD' Somatoform Symptom Disorder. Just to ensure that this category includes as many of us as possible, they have decided that

a) Even if you have a medical condition, you can still also suffer from SSD.

b) Even if you have no history which would be expected to lead to a psychiatric disorder, you can still suffer from SSD.

So you can be medically ill and have no history which would lead to a mental illness and still be classified as having a Somatic Symptom Disorder. You will not be surprised to learn that 'Chronic Fatigue Sydrome' is included within this category.

As of January, 2012 two footnotes can be added to this article.

According to a recent letter written by Professor Malcolm Hooper to Iain Duncan Smith, the current minister for work and pensions, that department classifies people with CFS/ME as having a psychiatric condition. This is illegal because the World Health Organisation categories are legally binding on the member of the EU, and the WHO classifies ME as a neurological disorder.

A detailed discussion of developments re WHO classification can be found at Suzy Chapman's website, www.meagenda.wordpress.com. (37)   The Twitter posts listed on the right of the page direct the reader to recent developments, including responses to the document below.

Regarding 'Somatic Symptom Disorder', The former head of the DSM 5 team, Dr. Allen J. Frances has written two articles which are highly critical of DSM 5, the second of which (DSM 5 In Distress, Mislabelling Medical Illness as a Mental Disorder) apologises for leaving SSD off the list of the ten major criticisms which are the subject of his first article and adds this incorrect labelling of people who have CFS/ME as the eleventh major fault. This article can be found   at   www.psychologytoday.com/blog/dsm5-in-distress/201212/mislabeling-medical-illness-mental-disorder. (38) Dr. Frances' suggestions have been rejected.

In this booklet, I've used the labels more or less randomly, as I know that many people labelled with CFS or its variants will be people who have ME. I am making the assumption that (whichever label they use) the psychiatrists will generally be referring a collection of people who may or may not have ME (for example, the subjects used in the PACE Trial, or in the reviews studied by Joyce, Hotopf and Wessely see below. (39)). The medical researchers (such as those whose work is listed in the references to the body of this book) appear to be describing patients who do suffer from ME.

The name-us.org website is very useful for historical records, and available downloads, especially the 2012 ICC Primer for Medical Practitioners.

Joyce, Hotopf and Wessely (39). In the section on 'Results, Characteristics of samples used', it states 'A wide variety of definitions of CF and CFS were used, and relatively few studies used operational criteria for CFS.'

AN EXAMPLE OF PSYCHIATRY THINK: PLAYING WITH STATISTICS!

In Joyce, Hotopf and Wessely (39), the authors find that 'the patient's belief in a physical cause of their symptoms ...predicted a poor outcome in every study in which it was measured.' The use of the term 'predictor', taken literally to mean something that 'speaks before' an event, would seem to imply that holding the belief is somehow part of what is causing the illness (an inference that the reader is clearly intended to make). This provides the rationale for their claim that ME/CFS can be 'reversed' simply by changing that belief: this is why Cognitive Behaviour Therapy plays such a major role in treatment regimes.

It does not seem to occur to these people that if you have been sick for a long time with a disabling illness, then 'believing' that it has a physical cause is a fairly rational response. Or, as Komaroff says in his review of the Manu's book on 'functional somatic' illnesses, *'if a person has a physical illness, it is not abnormal, neurotic or unrealistic to believe that they have a physical illness'* (3)

But statistics can be fun – let's have a shot at playing the statistics game:

We can do a hypothetical piece of research. Let us imagine that we conduct a survey of 100 people who have had an illness for twenty years. Our survey comprises a group of diabetics, a group of people with MS, a group of people who have had various forms of cancer over a period of twenty years, a group who have lupus, and a group of people with ME/CFS. To keep the math simple, let's say each group has twenty members.

Now we ask all of them whether they believe that they are suffering from a physical illness. 98 out of 100 believe that this is the case. (Let's say that two of the diabetics insist there's nothing wrong with them, and refuse to cooperate with treatment. Perhaps one of them subsequently dies, as not believing that you have a physical illness when you actually do doesn't always save you.)

As we know that 80 of our 100 do have an identified physical illness, *there is a high correlation between believing that one has a physical illness, and actually having one.*

'Believing one has a physical illness' has now become a 'predictor' of actually having one. So, since our people who have ME/CFS believe they have a physical illness, we are statistically persuaded that ME/CFs must be a physical illness.

(Those of you who are thinking 'cart before the horse', leave the room now! You heretics might even be imagining that there are better ways of figuring out whether an illness is 'physical'. Tsk.) For those of us who are still in the room – if, as the article appears to conclude, believing you have an illness is what causes it, should we start using CBT to persuade diabetics, cancer sufferers, people with MS and lupus that they don't really have any physical illnesses and stop offering them any other treatments?

PROVING IT'S NOT REALLY PHYSICAL, AND CERTAINLY NOT TERMINAL...

Joyce, Hotopf and Wessely (39) report that among the patients in the surveys they included in their review, there were only three deaths reported, two unrelated to ME/CFS and one suicide.

Similar research will have been done in the past, to 'prove' that smoking cigarettes does not cause health problems, let alone deaths. Look at a set of people who have smoked for five years. Do any of them have particular health problems? No. Are any of them dead? No. So smoking doesn't cause health problems, or death.

But now let's look at the records of 1,000 people who have died, separate the smokers from the non-smokers and then look at the age of death and the cause of death. Oh dear. The smokers died a lot younger and most of them died of lung cancer or congestive lung disease. Autopsies show blackened lungs and heart problems that are not usual in people of that young age, compared to the non-smoking group. Now it begins to look like smoking does make you sick and can be a cause of death. So now we've got warnings on the packets.

So, as indicated above, something similar has occurred in the case of ME/CFS. Joyce *et al* looked at the studies selected on the criteria described above. They found only two unrelated deaths and one suicide. It's not a 'terminal illness'.

However, a research project looking at the causes and ages of death in people who had ME/CFS (40) came up with a high percentage of deaths due to heart failure, cancer, and suicide. Obviously there was no connection to ME/CFS. Except that the people who had CFS died of heart failure an average of thirty years earlier than members of the general population. They were ten years younger in the case of deaths by cancer and ten years younger in the case of deaths by suicide.

Does smoking cause cancer/shorten lives? We know that it does. Does ME/CFS cause heart failure, cancer and suicide? You tell me.

I think it was Mark Twain who said 'There are lies, damned lies, and statistics.'

WHY ARE THE FINDINGS OF HEMORHEOLOGY IGNORED BY THE MEDICAL COMMUNITY?

Hemotology, the study of the chemical properties of blood, is a very important tool in both diagnosis and treatment of a wide range of disorders.

Hemorheology, the study of the physical properties of blood, is not included in medical textbooks, not taught in medical school, and therefore not made use of in medical practice.

The book 'Blood Viscosity Factors – The Missing Dimension in Modern Medicine' is Les's contribution toward ameliorating this situation, and contains information relevant to people with a number of chronic conditions, including ME, MS, and diabetes.

The fact that this whole area of research seems to be overlooked remains a mystery to me. The research methods used by hemorheologists are no less rigorous, their evidence no less 'scientific' than other work which wins easy acceptance within the medical journals and medical textbooks.

Les has presented the results of his research with ME patients at conferences, one-to-one conversations with leading figures, in medical journals, and to patient groups. Yet is it rarely cited, and often discounted, most often on the basis of very small studies which have not used his research protocol.

The recommendations in the 2012 ICC Primer include Omega 3 essential fatty acids from fish oil as a nutritional supplement, and the observation that '....anecdotal studies suggest some patients with normal blood counts improve in energy level, cognition, weakness and mood with mega B12 injections.'

Why 'anecdotal studies', when Les' extensive research is available? (However, note that he states that only B12 as hydroxocobalamin will be effective.)

Wessely is given a knighthood: the whole field of hemorheology is ignored. What has to happen for this to change?

FINALLY – MY VAIN HOPE!

I believe (and expect that absolutely no one will agree!) that if the findings of the immunologists, the people who study the signs and effects of inflammation implicated in ME, the researchers into mitochondria, the geneticists, and the hemorheologists could be put together, we would find that we had just about all the pieces of the jigsaw needed for seeing the whole picture of this complex disease. Will this ever happen?

BIBLIOGRAPHY

1. *Myalgic Encephamyalitis: A Baffling Syndrome With a Tragic Aftermath.* **Ramsay, Dr. A Melvin.** 1986.

2. **NHS National Institute for Health and Clinical Excellence.** CG53 Chronic Fatigue, Myalgic Encephalomyelitis. *www.nice.org.uk.* [Online] August 2007. [Cited: 3 August 2012.] Emphasis is on 'maintaining and if possible, gradually extending an individual's physical capacity'.

3. *Review of The Psychopathology of Functional Somatic Syndromes by Peter Manu.* **Komaroff, Anthony L. M.D.** 26, 2003 December 2004, New England Journal of Medicine, Vol. 351, pp. 2777-2778. Manu concludes that these disorders are not 'primary affective disorders'. K notes if illness is organic, it's not 'abnormal behaviour' to believe that it is. Also, 'somatoform' is never defined.

4. *International Consensus Criteria for ME (Myalgic Encephalomyelitis).* **Carruthers, BM, van de Sande, MI.** 20 July 2011, Journal of Internal Medicine. Recommends mmediate diagnosis, requires PENE (post exertional neuroimmune exhaustion) for diagnosis.

5. **Finlay, Sue.** An illlness doctors don't recognise. *The Observer.* 1 June 1986. The article that explained ME so I finally knew what my illness was. No definitive diagnostic test, no treatment, but you could get better if you rested..

6. **ME Association.** NHS specialist services throughout the UK. *ME Association.* [Online] [Cited: 10 August 2012.] Provides staff lists :Mostly psychiatrists, psychologists, OT's, Physio's, Rehab. http://www.meassocition.org.uk/?page_id=1382.

7. *A review on cognitive behavioral therapy (CBT) and graded exercise therapy (GET) in myalgic encephalomyelitis (ME)/chronic fatigue syndrome (CFS): CBT/GET is not only ineffective and not evidence-based, also potentially harmful for many ME/CFS patients.* **Twisk, F, Maes, M.** 3, 2009, Neuro Endocrinol Lett, Vol. 30, pp. 284-299. ME/CFS abnormalities: inflammation, immune dysfunction, oxidative and nitrosative stress, channelopathy, defective stress response mechanisms and a hypoactive hypothalamic-pituitary-adrenal axis. CBT/GET therefore unethical.

8. **Acheson, A D.** The clinical syndrome variously called benign myalgic encephalomyelitis, Iceland Disease and epidemic neuromyasthenia. [book auth.] Byron M Hyde and J A Goldstein. *The Clinical and Scientific Basis of Myalgic Encephalomyelitis/Chronic Fatigue Syndrome.* s.l. : The Nightingale Foundation, 1992. 'In the management of the acute phase, absolute rest provides

the best outcome' 'The association of premature rehabilitation with relapse is well described'.

9. **Simpson, Leslie O.** The Importance of Blood Flow and Evening Primrose Oil in ME. [ed.] Sandra Goodman Ph.D. *Positive Health PH Online.* April 2010:, 169.

10. **Simpson, LO and Blake, N.** *Ramsay's Disease - ME (Myalgic Encephalomyelitis) and the Unfortunate Creation of CFS.* s.l. : Lifelight Publishing, 2013. ISBN: 978-0-9571817-2-4.

11. **Simpson, Dr. L. O.** *Blood Viscosity Factors - The Missing Dimension to Modern Medicine.* Highlands : Mumford Institute. pp. 247-263. Important contribution to understanding symptoms of many chronic illnesses. ISBN: 978-0-615-25457-9.

12. *Nondiscocytic erythrocytes in myalgic encephalomyelitis.* **Simpson, LO.** 1989, New Zealand Medical Journal, pp. 102:106-7.

13. *Welcome to the Conference.* **Invest in ME.** 1, s.l. : UK Charity Invest in ME, 2012, Journal of Invest in ME, Vol. 6, pp. 3,4. Norwegian Government apologises to patients for treatment with CBT and GET.

14. **Simpson, LO.** *Questions Asked by ME Sufferers in Six Countries.* Dunedin : MEISS (Otago/Southland) Inc. Summary of Dr. Simpson's answers to questions asked by ME sufferers.

15. **Spotila, Jennie.** Exercise Testing and Results. *Occupy CFS.* [Online] Occupy CFS, 3 July 2012. [Cited: 5 September 2012.] Gives a very detailed explanation of

the role of reaching/exceeding anaerobic threshold in ME/CFS. http://www.occupycfs.com/exercise-testing-and-results.

16. *Patients with chronic fatigue syndrome performed worse than controls in a controlled repeated exercise study despite a normal oxidative phosphorylation capacity.* **Vermeulen, Ruud CS, et al., et al.** 93, 2010, Journal of Translational Medicine, Vol. 8.

17. *Talk given at Hull ME Group Meeting Graduate Medical School.* **Dowsett, Dr. Betty.** circa 1990. 'Save your energy for doing things you enjoy.'.

18. *Chronic fatigue syndrome: identifying zebras amongst the horses.* **Harvey SB, Wessely S.** 58, 2009, BMC Medicine, Vol. 7. Fig 1: their model of CFS 'Maintaining factors - behavioral/ deconditioning' illustrates the Wessely School beliefs.

19. *Is physical deconditioning a perpetuating factor in chronic fatigue syndrome? A controlled study on maximal exercise performance and relations with fatigue, impairment and physical activity.* **Bazelmans, E, Bleijenberg, G, Van der Meer, JWM, Folgering, H.** 16 January 2001, Cambridge Journals Online, Psychological Medicine, Vol. 31, p. 1070114. Results: There were no statistically significant differences in physical fitness between CFS patients and their controls. Nine CFS patients had a better fitness than their control. Conclusions: Physical deconditioning does not seem a perpetuating factor.

20. *Comparison of adaptive pacing therapy, cognitive behaviour therapy, graded exercise therapy, and specialist medical care for chronic fatigue syndrome (PACE): a randomised trial.* **White PD, Goldsmith KA, Johnson AL, Potts L, Walwyn R, DeCesare JC, Baber HL, Burgess, M, Clark LV, Cox DL, Bavinton J, Angus BJ, Murphy G, Murphy M, O'Dowd H, Wilks D, McCrone P, Chalter T, Sharpe M.** 5 March 2011, The Lancet, pp. 823-836. Using Oxford criteria, purports to indicate CBT and GET 'can safely' be added to Spec Med Care (SMC) to moderately improve outcomes for CFS; APT (pacing) not effective. (APT controlled by patient, CBT/GET controlled by professional) See Hooper critique..

21. *The Immunological Basis of ME/CFS: what is already known?* **Williams, Margaret.** 1, s.l. : The Charity Invest in ME, May 2012, The Journal of Invest in ME, Vol. 6, pp. 29-98. Compiliation of documented immune system abnormalities in ME/CFS from 1983-2011.

22. **Stout, Martha, Ph.D.** Inside the Mind of a Sociopath. [book auth.] Martha Stout. *The Sociopath Next Door: The Ruthless vx. the Rest of Us.* New York : Broadway Books, 2005.

23. *Organisational sociopaths: rarely challenged, often promoted. Why?* **Pech, Richard J, Slade, Bret W.** 3, s.l. : Emerald Group Publishing Limited, 2007, Society and Business Review, Vol. 2, pp. 254-269. Describes how management culture can lead to promotion of

sociopaths: manipulators and bullies who abuse power and victimise the vulnerable.

24. *Clinical and Research Updates in Myalgic Encephalomyelitis.* **Conference, 7th Invest in ME International ME/CFS.** London : Invest in ME, 2012.

25. **Wilson, Criona.** The Sophia Mirza Archive. *MEactionuk.* [Online] [Cited: 28 October 2012.] Account of life and death of Sophia Mirza, cause of death kidney failure due to ME/CFS, medical mistreatment..

26. *B-cell depletion therapy using Rituximab in ME/CFS.* **Fluge, Dr Oystein, Mella, Professor Olav.** London : UK Charity Invest in ME, 2012. 7th International ME/CFS Conference. Improvements/recovery using B-cell depletion therapy undermines psychiatric view, Norwegian Govt apologises.

27. **Hooper, Professor Malcolm.** Complaint to Editor of The Lancet about the PACE Trial Articles. *MEactionuk.* [Online] [Cited: 28 October 2012.] This is a lengthy and very systematic analysis of the flaws in the PACE Trial, which purported to show CBT and GET are 'safe' and 'effective', neither of which is true.

28. *Correspondence to Lancet re PACE.* **Kewley, A.J.** 17 May 2011, Lancet, pp. 1832-3. Change in assessment method, lack of objective data (actometer), small increase in walking distance compared to healthy elderly, only 41% reporting 'positive change'..

29. *Correspondence to Lancet re PACE.* **Kindlon, T.** 17 May 2011, Lancet, Vol. 377, p. 1833. Activities for CBT could have replaced other activity, so no total increase. Small increase in 6-min walking distance. Many reports of adverse reactions, biological reasons mean conclusion that these are 'safe' is premature.

30. *Why myalgic encephalomyelitis/chronic fatigue syndrome (ME/CFS) may kill you: disorders in the inflammatory and exidative and nitrosative stress (IO&NS) pathways may explain cardiovascular disorders in ME/CFS.* **Maes, M, Twisk, FN.** 6, 2009, Neuro Endocrinol Lett, Vol. 30, pp. 677-693.

31. Help filling out ESA 50. *www.nawra.org.uk.* [Online] [Cited: 29 October 2012.]

32. **Shropshire ME Group.** Hints for completing the ESA 50 form. *www.shropshiremegroup.org.* [Online] [Cited: 29 October 2012.] Useful advice for ME patient filling out ESA form.

33. *name-us.org.* [Online]

34. *Royal Free epidemic of 1955; a reconsideration.* **McEvedy, CP, Beard, AW.** 3 January 1970, British Medical Journal. Using notes including those of patients already dismissed as 'hysterical', concludes ME is a form of 'mass hysteria'. This view dominates medical and popular opinion right up to the present.

35. *Correspondence to Lancet re PACE.* **Feehan, S.M.** 17 May 2011, Lancet, pp. 1831-1832.

36. **Wessely, Professor Simon.** Death Threats to ME Researchers. [interv.] Tom Fielden. *Today.* s.l. : BBC, 2 August 2011. Wessely diverting attention from serious criticism of PACE by complaining about 'death threats' from ME people, claiming their objections were to the 'stigma' of a psychiatric diagnosis. .

37. **Chapman, Suzy.** *meagenda.wordpress.com.* [Online] Suzy Chapman runs a number of sites following developments of classification: DSM, ICD..

38. **Frances, Dr. Allen J.** DSM5 In Distress - Mislabelling Medical Illness Mental Disorder. *psychologytoday.com/blog/201212/dsm5-in-distress-mislabelling-medical-illness-mental-disorder.* [Online]

39. *The prognosis of chronic fatigue and chronic fatigue syndrome: a systematic review.* **Joyce J, Hotopf M, Wessely S.** London : s.n., 1997, Q J Med, Vol. 90, pp. 223-233. Because long-term severely ill patients often belonged to a self-help group and believed their illness to be organic, these are labelled 'predictors' of long-term illness. This becomes the justification for using CBT to change this belief.

40. *Causes of Death Among Patients With Chronic Fatigue Syndrome.* **Jason LA, Corradi K, Gress S, Williams S, Torres-Harding S.** 7, s.l. : Taylor & Francis Online, 2006, Health Care for Women International, Vol. 27, pp. 615-626. Main causes of death: heart failure (30 yrs younger than av), cancer, suicide, 10 years younger than av.

Lightning Source UK Ltd.
Milton Keynes UK
UKOW06f2254020916

281992UK00010BA/253/P